YOGA POSES TO DO WITH YOUR KIDS

AN ALL TIME GUIDE

KATE .P

Contents

CHAPTER ONE

INTRODUCTION

One of the best ways to encourage physical activity, mindfulness, and a stronger link between you and your children is to introduce yoga poses to them. Here's an enjoyable and easy yoga pose sequence that you can attempt together:

Aloha Pose (Mt. Pose):

Put your feet hip-width apart and stand tall.

Arms raised, palms facing one another.

Inhale deeply and imagine yourself firmly planted like a mountain.

Vrksasana, or Tree Pose:

Place your weight on one foot.

Position the opposing foot's sole on the standing leg's inner thigh or calf.

Cross your arms over like branches or bring your hands together at the middle of your chest.

Repeat on the other side.

Dog with Downward Gaze (Adho Mukha Svanasana):

With wrists under shoulders and knees under hips, begin on your hands and knees.

Raise your hips toward the ceiling and make an inverted V with your arms and legs straight.

Head relaxed between arms, heels pressed toward floor.

To stretch your hamstrings and calves, pedal your feet.

Stretching a cat-cow:

With wrists under shoulders and knees under hips, begin on your hands and knees.

Take a breath, raise your head, and arch your back (Cow Pose).

Exhale, curve your back, and bring your chin up to your chest (Cat Pose).

Continue, switching between the two stances with ease.

Bending into a butterfly (Baddha Konasana):

Bring the soles of your feet together while sitting on the floor, allowing your knees to drop to the sides.

Cling to the feet or ankles.

With your knees softly flapping up and down like butterfly wings, sit up straight.

Pose of the Child (Balasana):

With your big toes touching and your knees hip-width apart, drop to the floor.

Fold forward while sitting back on your heels and extend your arms in front of or next to your body.

Breathe deeply while placing your forehead on the ground.

The Ananda Balasana, or Happy Baby Pose:

With your legs drawn in toward your chest, lie on your back.

Stretch the knees apart from the torso while holding onto the outside borders of the feet.

Like a contented infant, gently sway from side to side.

Encourage your children to explore their bodies and take deep breaths while they play with these poses. By assuming the roles of animals or items associated with the poses, you can even turn it into a game. And never forget that the most crucial thing is to cherish the time you spend with your kids and help them develop a love of movement and mindfulness.

Yoga's importance for kids

Children who practice yoga can get several mental and physical health benefits. The following are some main arguments in favor of yoga for kids:

Physical Condition:

enhances coordination, balance, and flexibility.

fortifies bones and muscles.

encourages appropriate alignment and posture.

increases endurance and general physical fitness.

Controlling Emotions:

teaches self-awareness and mindfulness.

aids with children's stress and anxiety management.

promotes serenity and relaxation.

offers coping mechanisms for handling emotions.

Cognitive Growth:

increases focus and concentration.

enhances cognitive and memory performance.

encourages imagination and creativity.

enhances the ability to solve problems.

Social Competencies:

encourages a feeling of belonging and community.

encourages compassion and understanding for others.

promotes cooperation and teamwork in pair or group postures.

increases the ability to communicate through encounters and verbal cues.

Understanding and Accepting Your Body:

aids in children's increased awareness of their own body and feelings.

promotes acceptance of oneself and an appreciation of one's special talents.

encourages confidence in oneself and a healthy body image.

wholesome behaviors

fosters awareness of one's eating patterns and dietary preferences.

promotes consistent exercise and physical activity.

encourages the use of relaxation techniques before bed and improved sleep habits.

Wholesome Well-Being:

teaches youngsters coping skills and good behaviors that will serve them well into life.

gives resources for handling the responsibilities and pressures of everyday living.

lays the groundwork for a lifetime enjoyment of mindfulness, exercise, and self-care.

All things considered, yoga provides kids with a comprehensive approach to health, addressing mental, emotional, and physical elements of wellbeing. Children can acquire abilities and routines that support resilience and well-being throughout their lives by practicing yoga from an early age.

Family yoga practice has several advantages.

There are several advantages to practicing yoga as a family, both personally and socially. Here are a few benefits:

Yoga sessions offer a serene and harmonious setting for family members to spend quality time together, fostering bonding and connection. Family ties can be strengthened and relationships amongst family members can be strengthened by sharing this experience.

Better Communication: Doing yoga with one another promotes candid dialogue and support from one another. It fosters empathy and understanding by providing a safe area for family members to express their ideas, emotions, and experiences.

Physical Well-Being: There are several physical health advantages to yoga, such as improved flexibility, strength, and balance. All members of the family benefit from general health and wellbeing when they practice yoga together.

Emotional Well-Being: Stress, anxiety, and depression can be lessened by incorporating mindfulness and meditation techniques into yoga. Family members can help one other manage emotions and become more emotionally resilient by doing yoga together.

Cooperation and teamwork are essential for partner and group yoga postures, which foster family members' cooperation and teamwork. Posing together promotes a sense of oneness as well as encouragement and support for one another.

Positive Role Modeling: Yoga-practicing parents who put their health and wellbeing first provide a good example for their kids. Parents can impart healthy habits and ideals that can last a lifetime on their children's lifestyles by practicing yoga as a family.

Respect for Culture: The philosophy and culture of ancient India are the origins of yoga. Families can receive the chance to understand and respect various cultures and customs by doing yoga together.

Yoga promotes attention and being in the present moment by teaching these two concepts. A shared sense of mindfulness and present is fostered by family yoga, which enables members to connect more fully with one another and with themselves.

Yoga lessons may be lively and imaginative, particularly when done with younger students. Family yoga sessions are engaging and entertaining for all participants because they frequently include games, storytelling, and creative positions.

Long-Term Health Benefits: Starting a regular yoga practice as a family can have a positive impact on everyone's quality of life in the long run by lowering the likelihood of developing chronic illnesses and boosting immunity.

In general, family yoga practice offers a comprehensive approach to health and wellbeing, nourishing the body, mind, and spirit while fortifying ties within the family and promoting a sense of oneness and connection.

Exercises to Warm Up

Whether you're doing yoga, playing sports, or any other physical activity, it's imperative to warm up your body and mind beforehand. The following are some efficient warm-up exercises that can be used by people of all ages and fitness levels:

Joint rotations: To improve joint lubrication and mobility, gently rotate key joints in circular motions, including the wrists, elbows, shoulders, neck, hips, knees, and ankles.

Dynamic Stretching: Make stretches that are similar to the movements you'll be making throughout the main exercise. Walking lunges, arm and leg swings, and torso twists are a few examples.

Sun Salutations (Surya Namaskar): Sun Salutations are a great way to warm up for yoga since they gradually engage the entire body and increase blood flow.

Jumping Jacks: This age-old exercise works all major muscle groups, elevates the heart rate, and improves circulation it's a terrific way to warm up your entire body.

High Knees and Butt Kicks: To warm up your leg muscles and increase flexibility, alternately raise your knees toward your chest and your heels toward your buttocks while you march or jog in place.

Arm Circles: To warm up your shoulder muscles, stand with your arms outstretched parallel to the floor. Then, slowly increase the size of your arm circles.

CHAPTER TWO

Hip Circles: To warm up your lower back and hip joints, stand with your feet hip-width apart and your hands on your hips. Then, move your hips in a circle, first in one direction and then the other.

Core Activation: To engage the core muscles and support the spine, try activities like planks, bird-dogs, or light crunches.

Challenges with balance: Engage in balancing activities that enhance proprioception and stability, such as standing on one leg or doing yoga positions.

Breathing techniques: To relax the mind, enhance oxygen intake, and direct attention inward, incorporate deep breathing techniques like diaphragmatic breathing or alternate nostril breathing.

To prevent strain or injury, always remember to modify the warm-up exercises to the individual needs and capabilities of the participants and to progressively raise the intensity. Usually lasting five to ten minutes, warm-ups aim to prepare the body for more demanding action by progressively raising body temperature, heart rate, and circulation.

The following typical yoga positions are appropriate for all skill levels:

Aloha Pose (Mt. Pose):

Place your feet together or hip-width apart and stand tall.

Tighten your thighs, raise your chest, and let your shoulders drop.

With palms facing front, the arms are at the sides.

As you hold the pose, concentrate on taking deep breaths and establishing your footing.

Dog (Adho Mukha Svanasana) facing downward:

Commence in the tabletop posture, hands and knees.

Raise your hips and extend your arms and legs straight.

Form the body into an inverted V form.

To stretch the spine, press the palms and heels toward the ground.

(Virabhadrasana I): Warrior I

Take a single step back while standing.

Maintaining the front knee precisely over the ankle, bend it at a 90-degree angle.

Put your hands up, palms facing each other, and square your hips forward.

Maintain a powerful, straight back leg while pressing the foot's outside edge into the mat.

Vrksasana, or Tree Pose:

Put your feet hip-width apart and stand tall.

Place the sole of the other foot against the inside thigh or calf (avoid the knee) while you shift weight onto one foot and elevate the other.

Raise your hands in a prayer position above your head or to the chest.

To help with stability and balance, identify a focus point.

Pose of the Child (Balasana):

With your big toes touching and your knees slightly wider than hip width apart, kneel on the mat.

Folding forward, extend your arms in front of you or rest them by your sides, sit back into your heels.

Lay your forehead down on the mat and take a deep breath. Then, focus on relaxing your entire body.

Cat-Cow Pose (also known as Marjaryasana-Bitilasana):

Begin in the tabletop position, hands and knees, with your spine in a neutral position.

Taking a deep breath, raise your head and tailbone toward the ceiling while arching your back (cow position).

Let out a breath, arch your back, tuck your chin into your chest, and tuck your tailbone under (cat position).

Move between these two positions while keeping your breathing and movement in rhythm.

Forward Fold in Sitting (Paschimottanasana):

With your legs out in front of you, sit on the mat.

Take a breath, extend your back, and release it as you bend forward at the hips.

Maintain a long spine while reaching toward the thighs, shins, or feet.

Breathe deeply into the stretch while letting your head and neck relax.

Head to toes (Savasana):

With your legs outstretched and your arms by your sides, palms facing up, assume a flat back position.

Shut your eyes and let go of all tension in your body, allowing your muscles to become softer.

To revitalize the body and mind, stay in the pose for a few minutes while concentrating on deep, conscious breathing.

As practitioners advance in their yoga journey, there are innumerable variations and adaptations to try out. These positions are only a starting point. Always pay attention to your body, take deep breaths, and approach your practice with awareness and mindfulness.

Calm down and unwind

A yoga practice must include cool-down and relaxation to help the body and mind shift from an active state to one of rest and recuperation. Incorporate the following relaxing techniques and cool-down positions into your yoga practice:

Bending Forward While Seated (Paschimottanasana):

With your legs out in front of you, sit on the mat.

Breathe in to stretch the spine; exhale to fold forward and hinge at the hips.

Head and neck should be relaxed when you reach for the thighs, shins, or feet.

For several breaths, hold the posture, concentrating on deep breathing and letting go of any tension in your hamstrings and back.

Spinal Twist in Supine:

Assume a T-position while lying on your back with your arms out to the sides.

With the foot on the other side of the mat, bend one knee and cross it across the torso.

Try to maintain both shoulders grounded by turning the head in the opposite direction of the bowed knee.

CHAPTER THREE

After holding the twist for a few breaths, switch sides.

Viparita Karani's song "Legs Up the Wall":

Place one hip against the wall as you sit close to it.

Lying back on the mat, make an L-shape with your body, and swing your legs up the wall.

Shut your eyes, put your arms at your sides with your palms facing up, and concentrate on taking deep, belly breaths.

For five to ten minutes, hold this stance to increase circulation and induce calm.

Bound Angle Pose in Reclining (Supta Baddha Konasana):

With your feet together and your knees bent, lie on your back and let them drop to the sides.

Put your other hand on your heart and your first on your belly.

Shut your eyes and concentrate on taking deep, rhythmic breaths. As you breathe in and out, feel your tummy rise and fall.

Take a few minutes to remain in this pose so that your body can open and relax.

Head to toes (Savasana):

With your legs outstretched and your arms by your sides, palms facing up, assume a flat back position.

Shut your eyes and let go of all stress in your body, from head to toe.

Pay attention to your breathing and the way that your inhalations and exhalations naturally occur.

Spend five to ten minutes in savasana, giving up all thoughts and anxieties and just giving yourself over to the present moment.

Relaxation with guidance or Yoga Nidra:

In order to achieve deep relaxation and rejuvenation, try a guided relaxation or Yoga Nidra session, where a teacher walks you through a methodical relaxation approach while emphasizing different body areas and breath awareness.

After your yoga practice, use these cool-down poses and relaxation practices to support your mental, physical, and emotional well-being. This will help you leave the mat feeling thoroughly rested, rejuvenated, and refreshed.

Summary

In conclusion, there are numerous advantages to practicing yoga as a family that go beyond the physical aspects of the discipline. It is an effective means of fortifying ties within families, encouraging dialogue, and advancing general wellbeing in people of all ages. Families can strengthen their relationships and foster harmony and togetherness in the home by supporting one other's physical, mental, and emotional well-being through combined yoga sessions.

Yoga offers a comprehensive approach to wellness that takes into account the mind, spirit, and body. Families can benefit from increased flexibility, strength, and balance as well as important life lessons in self-awareness, stress reduction, and mindfulness by practicing yoga together. Additionally, doing yoga together as a family creates a positive atmosphere where people can support and encourage one another, strengthening bonds and making enduring memories.

Yoga gives families a place to gather, appreciate one another's strengths, and face life's obstacles with grace and resiliency—whether through energetic sequences, partner postures, or relaxation techniques. Families can enrich their lives both on and off the mat by embracing yoga as a shared activity and going on a path of self-discovery, growth, and connection.

Essentially, practicing yoga alone is not enough; it's a journey that takes on much greater significance when shared with others you hold dear. Families establish the groundwork for a better, happier, and more peaceful existence together as they join together to practice yoga and breathe, move, and explore the depths of their being.

THE END